Carrie and Larry

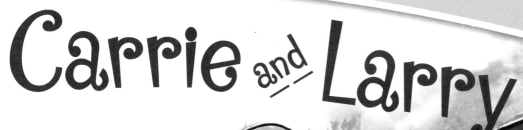

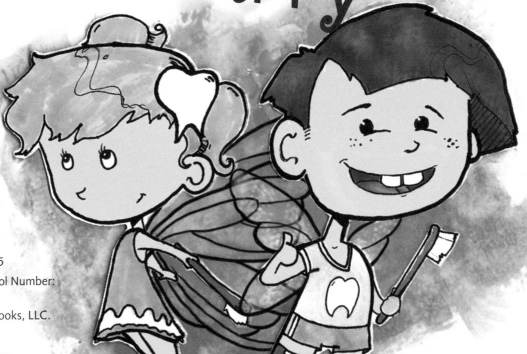

ISBN: 978-0-9833194-0-5

Library of Congress Control Number:
2015912737

Published by Babytooth Books, LLC.

Printed in the U.S.A.

CPSIA Compliance Information:
Job #129185
March / 2011
Reprint August / 2015

For further information contact Colorwise, Inc.
1125 Northmeadow Pkwy Suite 130
Roswell, GA 30076

THE Tooth-Tickling Fairies

About the Author

Dr. Michelle is married and has three children. The story of Carrie and Larry the Tooth-Tickling Fairies, was created to help educate parents about how to care for your child's teeth at home, beginning with the very first tooth. Often times, children either don't have easy access to dental care or they don't see a dentist until the age of four or five. This book makes dental care fun! Dr. Michelle's mission is to build a community valuing prevention, early detection and treatment of dental disease in children.

EDUCATION AND CERTIFICATIONS

Diplomate, the American Board of Pediatric Dentistry

Masters of Science in Dentistry, 2003, Indiana University

School of Dentistry DDS degree, 2001, Indiana University School of Dentistry

BA in psychology from the University of South Carolina

PROFESSIONAL ORGANIZATIONS

- Fellow Member, The American Academy of Pediatric Dentistry
- American Dental Association
- Indiana Society of Pediatric Dentistry

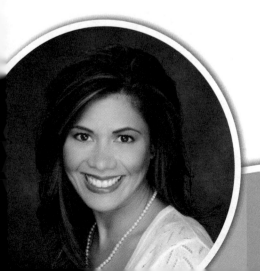

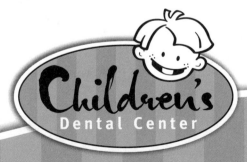

www.BabyToothCenter.com

Michelle H. Edwards, DDS, MSD

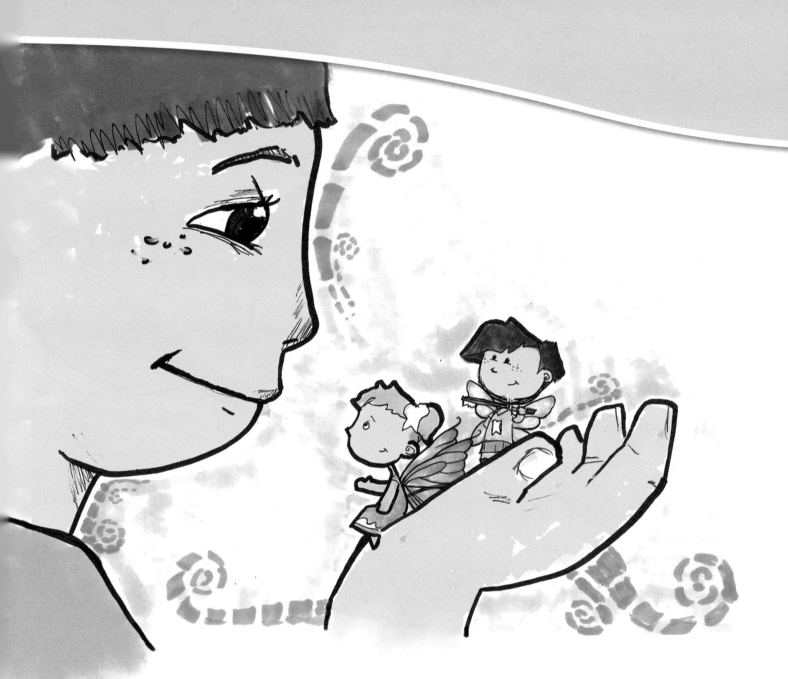

Carrie and Larry the Tooth-Tickling Fairies want to show you how to keep your teeth feeling merry!

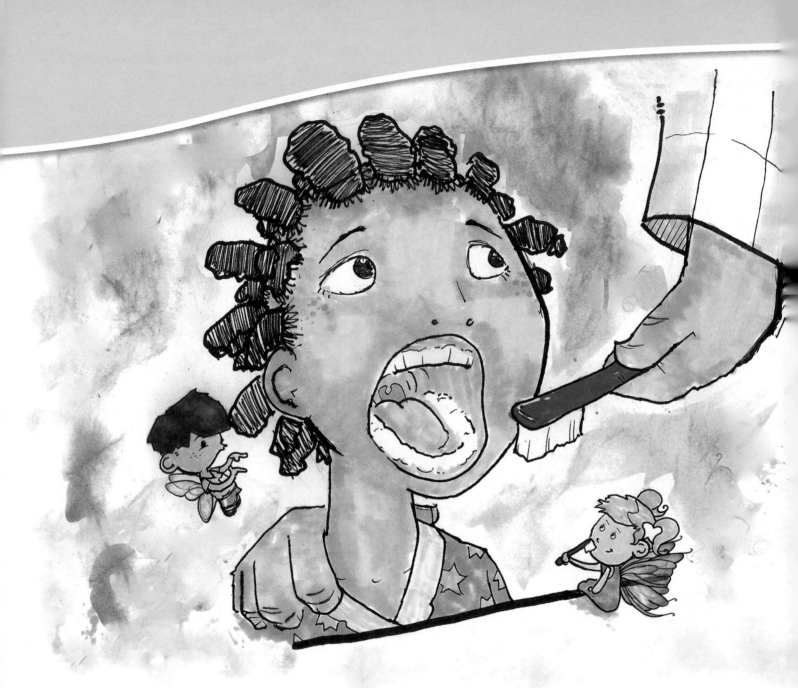

It is good to brush both morning and night and
floss through the teeth that are touching so tight.

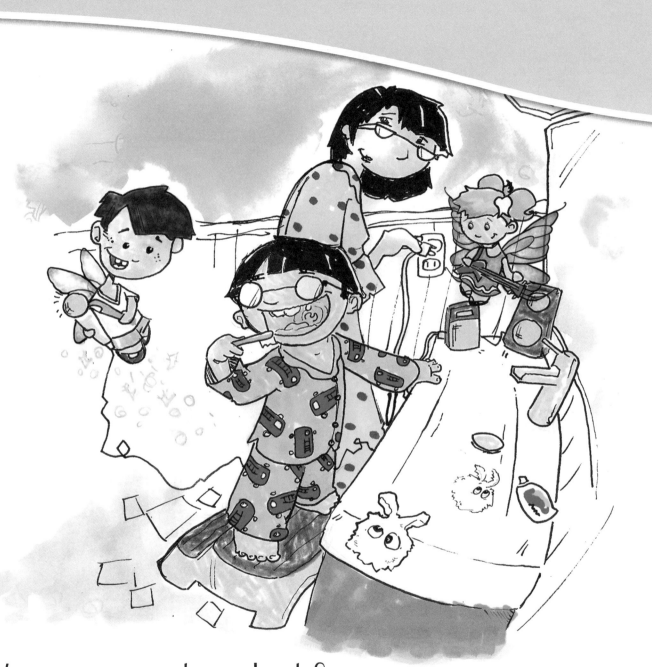

We sing a song to make it fun.
It makes all the sugar bunnies run!

(sung to 'Wheels on the Bus')

It goes, "This is the way we brush our teeth,
brush our teeth, brush our teeth.
This is the way we brush our teeth,
before we greet the sun.
Up and down and round and round.
Back and forth we go.
This is the way we brush our teeth
before we greet the sun."

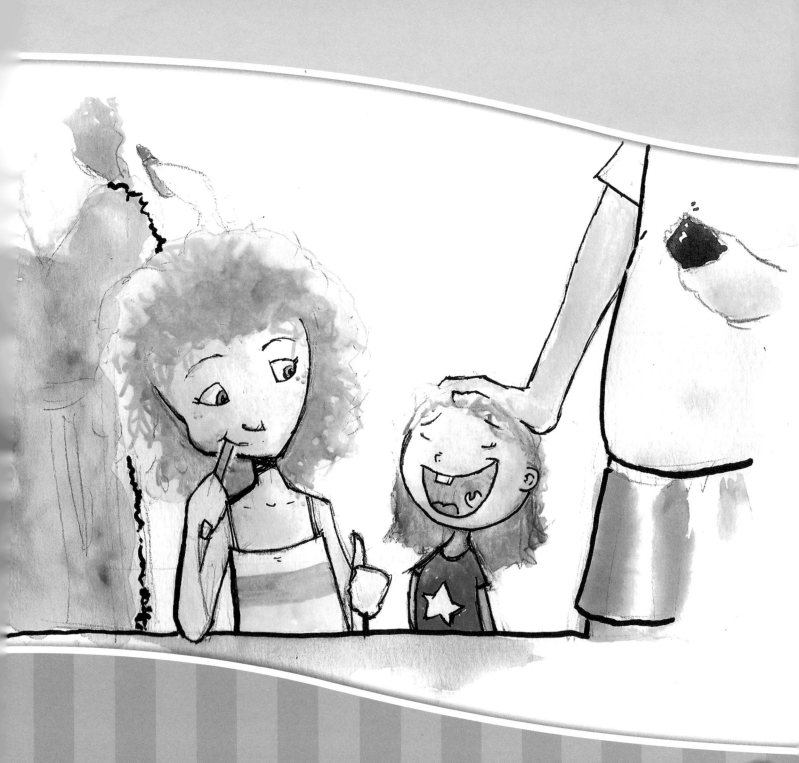

And again, at night...

"This is the way we brush our teeth,
brush our teeth, brush our teeth.
This is the way we brush our teeth,
before we go to bed.
Up and down and round and round.
Back and forth we go.
This is the way we brush our teeth
before we go to bed."

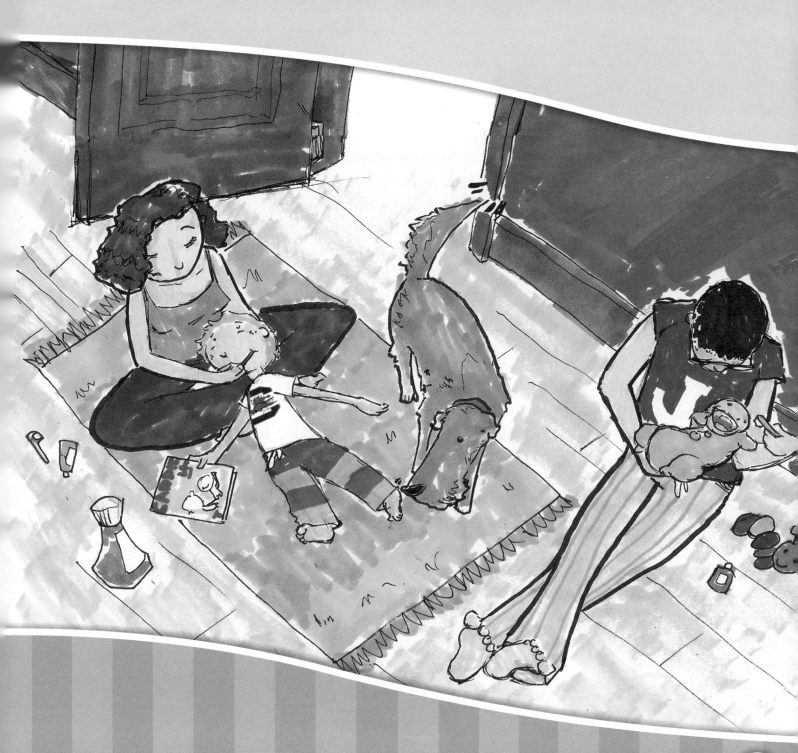

Back to Brush™

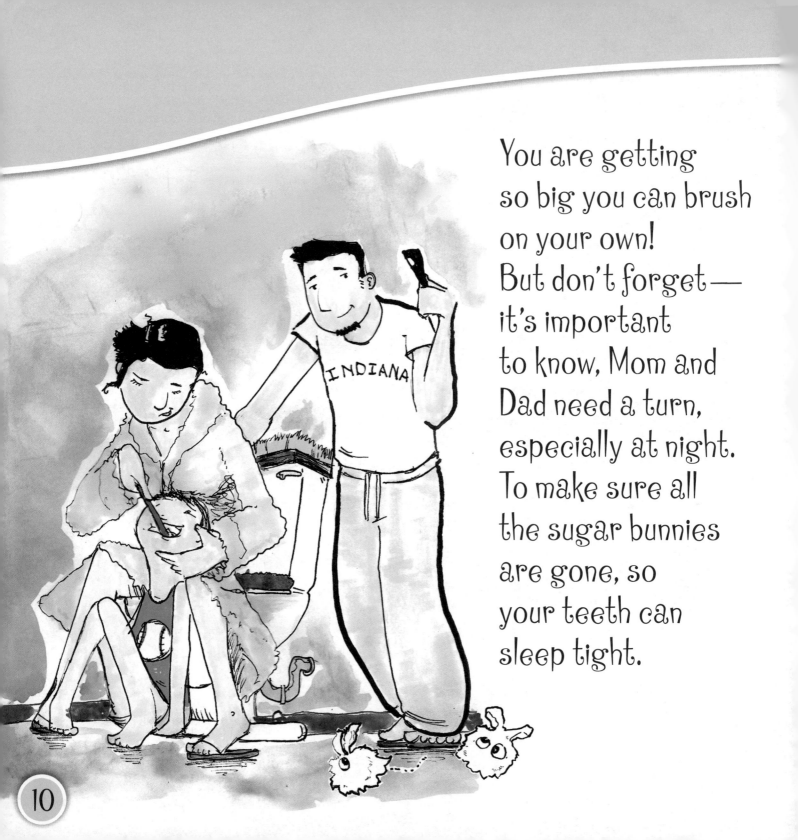

You are getting
so big you can brush
on your own!
But don't forget—
it's important
to know, Mom and
Dad need a turn,
especially at night.
To make sure all
the sugar bunnies
are gone, so
your teeth can
sleep tight.

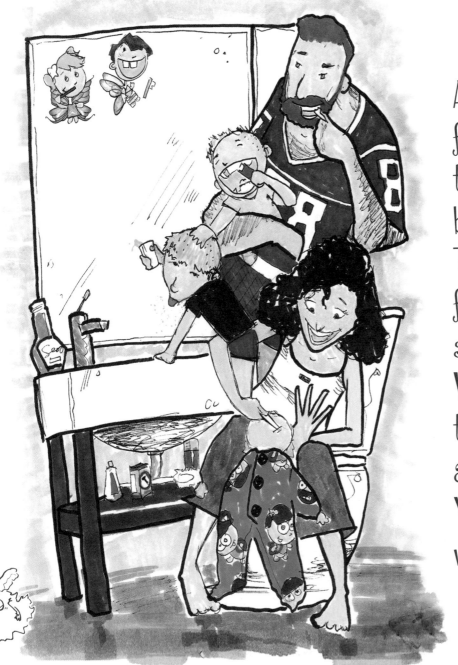

As tooth tickling
fairies, our job is
to watch from the
bathroom mirror!
To see the brushing,
flossing and spitting
so much clearer!
We love to tickle
teeth until they
are sparkling clean.
You can do it, if we
work as a team!

Raise Healthy Smiles

The American Academy of Pediatric Dentistry has recommended that children visit a dentist by their first birthday or 6 months after the first tooth comes in. Establishing a dental home for children at a very young age can provide preventive care beginning with a child's first tooth.

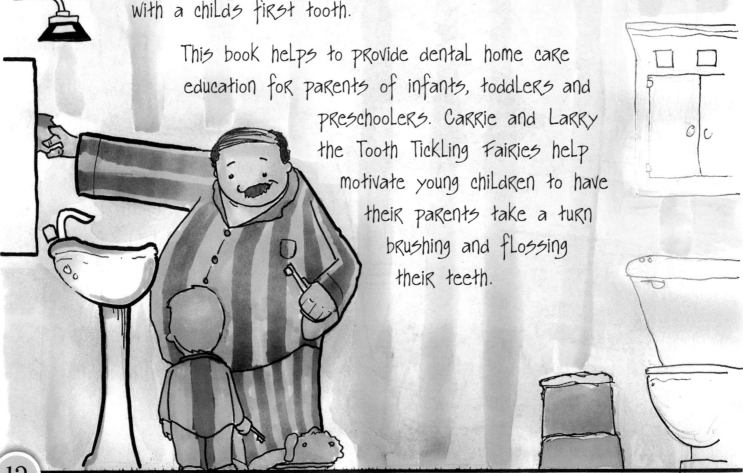

This book helps to provide dental home care education for parents of infants, toddlers and preschoolers. Carrie and Larry the Tooth Tickling Fairies help motivate young children to have their parents take a turn brushing and flossing their teeth.

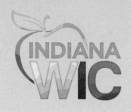

Let's work together to raise healthy children!

Here are a few things to remember to keep your child's mouth clean and healthy.

Babies:
Breastfeeding is best for mom and baby's health. Remember to wipe your baby's teeth off after feeding! Never put your baby to bed with a bottle or sippy cup of milk, juice, formula, or soda. If your baby takes a bottle before bed, wipe their teeth off with a baby washcloth. If the baby has back teeth, use a toothbrush.

Toddlers, Preschoolers and Young Children:
Choose foods and drink from the "DO" list and limit food and drinks from the "DON'T" list. Brush your child's teeth before bed. Introduce flossing when teeth are touching together. Here is a list of simple food swaps to keep your children's smiles healthy and beautiful!

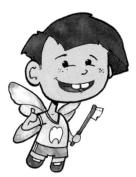

"DO" EAT THIS!	"DON'T" EAT THIS!
White milk	Juice – no more than 4 oz. a day
Chewable Vitamins	Gummy vitamins
Fresh fruit and vegetables	Gummy fruit snacks and candy
Cheese	Raisins
Water	Sports drinks
Crackers or pretzels	Potato chips
Yogurt	Ice cream
Cooked or whole grain cereal and bread	Dry sugary cereal
Tortillas	Tortilla chips

Tooth Tips for Tots

Following these simple tooth tips will help prevent dental decay in young children. It will also help reduce the amount of dental treatment a child will need in the long run.

1. See your pediatric dentist every 6 months starting by the age of one. Going to the dentist this early will allow your child to get acquainted with the dental surroundings and the dentist.

2. Brush teeth at least 2 times a day, especially before bed. When you sleep, your mouth is dry. When your mouth is dry, it is a breeding ground for dental decay. This is why going to bed with milk, juice, or any other drink is not good for your teeth.

3 Establish a tooth-brushing-time routine. Find a routine that works for you. Our personal routine at home is bath time, brush time, book time, bed time.

4 Technique is very important. The **Back to Brush**™ technique is illustrated on pages 9, 10, and 11. Having your child lay back while brushing has these advantages:

- You have more control. The child's head isn't bobbing around and you don't risk gagging them. The last molar on the chewing surface, top and bottom, is a hot spot for cavities— direct vision is very helpful in cleaning those areas.

- A child's facial muscles relax a bit when they are laying back and you can gently move their cheeks around to access all sides of their teeth.

- Have a flosser stick or floss ready and use it after brushing.

5 Aim the toothbrush at a 45 degree angle toward the gum line and brush in little circles. Wherever you are brushing in the mouth, aim for the gum line. The goal being to disrupt the plaque that forms on teeth.

6 Remember to floss where teeth are touching together. Another hot spot for cavities in children are between the last two teeth in the mouth—the molars.

7 Water is the best drink for sipping during the day and to take to bed at night.

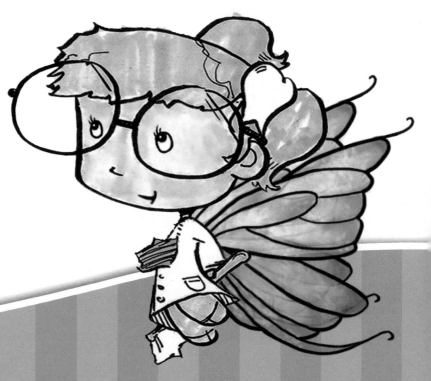

8 Limit juice to 4 oz. a day and drink it with meals. Eating gets the saliva going to help reduce the risk of cavities.